HERBS TO SOOTHE YOUR NERVES

These herbal remedies for stress and strain act on the blood, metabolism and all life processes, of which the nerves are an integral part. Thus they are capable of bringing a person's nervous system into harmony and health.

HERBS TO
SOOTHE YOUR NERVES

by
SARAH BECKETT

Drawings by Jill Fry

THORSONS PUBLISHERS LIMITED
Wellingborough, Northamptonshire

First published 1972
Second Impression 1975
Third Impression 1977

ISBN 0 7225 0209 5

Typeset by
Specialised Offset Services Limited, Liverpool
Made and Printed in Great Britain by
Weatherby Woolnough, Wellingborough, Northamptonshire

CONTENTS

INTRODUCTION

'A lesson in each flower,
A story in each tree and bower.
In every herb on which we tread
Are written words, which rightly read
Will lead us from earth's fragrant sod
To hope, and holiness to God.'
From an old herbal.

This book has been a joy to write for two reasons.

Firstly, it is good to write about something in which one has absolute faith, the natural herbs, put on earth for man when the world began and used to this day. Each little herbal plant, however insignificant, can bring help when prescribed correctly, to people suffering from all the many diseases to which man is heir. But that is not all. Herbs do their work gently and leave no side effects, and soon after commencing treatment it is not unusual to hear, 'I am beginning to feel better'. This is encouraging to both the patient and prescriber.

And secondly, it is hoped that numbers of people will read this small book who have never given much thought to anything but orthodox medicine. If the following pages are read, and food for thought is given to newcomers to herbal treatment, then it is possible that more men and women will turn away from drugs and reap the benefit of natural remedies.

Sarah Beckett.

ABOUT THE NERVOUS SYSTEM

In these days of stress and strain there is a great increase in the number of people suffering from nervous disorders of one kind or another. This is confirmed by the quantities of tranquillizers and sedatives prescribed. These give temporary relief in some cases, but they are palliative rather than curative as they do nothing towards building up the nervous system.

It is important to realize that sufferers from nervous complaints *are* really ill and need just as much treatment as people exhibiting physical symptoms. Patience should be exercised by family and friends; the complaint can be very trying and often there are few really concrete symptoms with which to deal.

Nervous tension and strain can lead to many symptoms, one of the most common takes the form of great anxiety about unimportant matters. The danger lies not in considering their problems rationally, but in allowing them to get magnified out of all proportion.

People often become very depressed but cannot give one good reason why this is so. Fears of various kinds creep in to torment the victim.

If is difficult to assess the depths to which shock or trauma penetrates. How often one hears of nervous troubles following the death of husband, wife or near relative; bad news is always a shock to, and strain on, the nervous system. Accidents also have a detrimental effect on the nerves and we have all heard the remark, 'He has never been the same since his car accident'.

Symptoms such as sleeplessness, nervous headache, anxiety, indigestion etc., may develop after shock, and unless the *cause* is dealt with correctly, the symptoms, whatever they may be, cannot be eliminated.

Similarly, it is not uncommon to meet patients who complain of a symptom — it may be palpitation, constipation, laryngitis, very often indigestion or stomach pains, and on questioning them it is found that the *cause* is worry, overtiredness or nervous tension. Again, by treating the cause, the physical symptoms, whatever they may be, disappear. To treat palpitation, constipation or laryngitis would merely palliate the condition.

A case comes to mind of a farmer who, after a very bad cold one winter, lost his voice and for weeks this troubled him; it would return to almost normal and then go again although the cold had cleared up completely. He was treated for laryngitis at the beginning without any results but on going deeper into his case, it was revealed that his wife had died very suddenly three months prior to this trouble. After having treatment for grief and his nervous system, his voice returned and he felt extremely well.

A young mother had her second baby when the first child was eighteen months old, and about three months afterwards she had a very itchy skin rash on her face and arms. This girl had a great deal on her hands and she was an 'anxious type' and it was realized that her nervous system needed the treatment and not her skin. After two months, not only was her skin without a blemish, but she felt very much better in herself and more able to cope with her family life.

Business men often get to the verge of a nervous breakdown through overwork and worry. Many women are similarly affected by the usual everyday stresses and strains but in addition, childbearing often has a profound effect on the nervous system both before and after *the* event. Another particularly difficult time is the menopause when nervous troubles often develop.

Herbs are capable of helping all kinds of nervous disorders but each case must be investigated individually, and the cause found if possible, in order that the correct prescription may be made.

HOW HERBS CAN HEAL

'Happy the age of which we moderns give
The name of "golden"; when men chose to live
On woodland fruits; and for their medicines took
Herbs from the field, and Simples from the brook.'

Ovid.

Hippocrates, who is recognized as the 'Father of Medicine' and who lived about the fourth century before

Christ, recorded in his writings the use of herbs in the treatment of disease.

Pliny, who lived about two thousand years ago, wrote: 'Hippocrates verely had this honour above all men, that hee was the first who wrote with the most perspicuitic of Physicke, and reduced the precepts and rules thereof into the bodie of an art; howbeit in all his books we find no other recipes but herbs.'

In A.D. 1490 there was a physician in Germany named William Bombast von Hohemhein. His son Theophratus was educated and sent to the same school as his father, but he soon became dissatisfied and went to work in the mines at Tyrol. He was fascinated by what he saw; minerals being purified by other minerals, and an idea came to him that he could purify human bodies in the same way. He began giving his patients minerals as medicines, but no records were kept so results of these experiments are not known.

From what we can gather he got very swollen headed and called himself Paracelsus, the reason is not given, and it is said that he publicly burned all the old books of Galen and Hippocrates and discarded all their ideas. He continued to use minerals in place of herbs, roots and barks.

Paracelsus died at the age of 50, and after his death there were hundreds of people who followed his method of treatment. From that has developed the system of allopathic medicine most widely used today.

Our present herbalists are followers of Galen and Hippocrates.

Herbs can help man to recover from the many and varied nervous conditions so prevalent today. They are gentle and soothing in action, safe, non-suppresive and have no side effects.

Most herbs contain substances which have a profound effect on the whole economy of man, the blood, the metabolism and all the processes vital to life.

Herbs are foods as well as medicines; they contain vitamins, starches, sugars, oils and other essential ingredients, and these are all synthesized according to nature, for the benefit of man.

During more recent times chemists have endeavoured to improve upon nature by isolating what they believe to be the active principle of various plants and making medicines from them. But experience has proved that these preparations do not have the same effect, nor do they give such satisfactory results as remedies prepared according to herbal principles. Then the whole herb, or the part containing the healing agent such as the root, leaves or flowers, is used as a whole and either boiled or infused (as tea is made), or cold water added. Specific instructions are given in each case and *all* the healing properties of the herb are taken into the system, to help the body as a whole return to normal.

The number of people taking tranquillizers today is legion. Those who seek an alternative, because they realize the dangers of drugs, can turn to herbs with confidence that they will be helped.

At the commencement of treatment, when herbal remedies are prescribed, tranquillizers may still be taken, but as the herbs build up the nervous system, they (the tranquillizers) will be relied upon less and less until finally they can be discontinued.

Remember — herbs act on the whole of the economy, of which the nerves are an integral part; thus they are capable of bringing the nervous system, and the patient, into harmony and health.

BALM
(*Melissa officinalis*)

'. . . Here liquors cast in fitting sort,
Of bruised Bawme and more base Honeywort.'
Virgil.

Also known as Sweet Balm, Lemon Balm, Honey Plant, Cure-All. The old herbalists knew it as Bawm.
Description: This is a common plant which often grows

in cottage gardens, and had its origin in the wild 'bastard balm', growing in woods, especially in southern England. The leaves grow opposite, are dark green, serrate and wrinkled. Small white flowers are very near the stem. It has a taste and odour like lemon. Gerard wrote, 'Our common Bawne having square stalks and blackish leaves, of a pleasant smell drawing near in smell and savour unto Citron . . . '

Part used: Whole herb.

The name balm is an abbreviation of balsam which signifies 'the chief of sweet-smelling oils' and in Hebrew it is known as *Bal-Smin*, 'Chief of Oils'. The botanical suffix *melissa* refers to the large quantity of honey (mel) contained in the flowers of this herb.

Pliny said, 'It is profitable planted where bees are kept, the hives should be rubbed with the leaves so causing the bees to keep together and others to come to them.'

This herb is especially valuable in nervous diseases and hysteria and is said to drive away 'all troublesome cares and thoughts out of the mind from melancholy . . .' — *Culpeper.*

The London Dispensary of 1969 said, 'The essence of balm given in Canary wine every morning will renew youth, strengthen the brain, relieve languishing nature and prevent baldness.'

John Evelyn said, 'Balm is sovereign for the brain, strengthening the memory and powerfully chasing away melancholy.'

'Bawn', say the Arabians, 'make the heart merry and joyful.'

It is said that John Jussey of Sydenham, who lived to the age of 116 years, breakfasted for fifty years on balm tea sweetened with honey.

Paracelsus believed that balm would completely revivify man.

The leaves used to be placed in ale and wine to impart their flavour and were thought to be restorative in the same way that balm 'tea' was drunk in the cottager's homes.

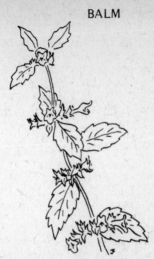

Balm

In Tudor times the juice was extracted from the leaves for wine making and it was used to rub on furniture to impart its lemony scent.

It is evident from the foregoing that balm can help people who get worked up to the point of feeling hysterical, and those who are depressed or have a bad memory.

It has a calming effect on the nervous system and helps the body to relax. It seems to bring fresh life to an over-tired system.

As a tea, balm is delicious and if taken at night it relieves tension and sleep is assured. If on the other hand balm tea is taken first thing in the morning it refreshes and any tiredness is swept away.

Directions for use: An infusion is made by pouring 1 pint of cold water on to 1 oz of the herb which should be left to stand for twelve hours. This should then be strained and a wineglassful taken three times daily. By infusing with cold water the volatile aromatic virtues are not dispelled by heat.

To make balm tea put a teaspoonful of the herb into a cup and add boiling water. This should be steeped for ten minutes before drinking.

BLACK COHOSH
(*Cimicifuga racemosa*)

'The powre of herbes, both which can hurt and ease
And which be wont t'enrange the restless sheepe.
And which be wont to work eternal sleepe.'

Spenser.

Also known as Black snakeroot, Bugbane, Rattleroot, Rattleweed, Squawroot.

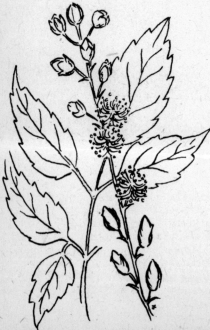

Black Cohosh

Description: Black cohosh grows in herbaceous borders so long as it has plenty of sunshine, but its home is America, Canada, and Kashmir. It has snake-like cream flowers — and the root is thick, hard and knotty with short lateral branches.

Part used: The root.

This herb has a marked influence on the nervous structures and should be given for the relief of insomnia and headaches with pain at the base of the brain and the back of the head.

Black cohosh has relaxing properties and is of excellent service in nervous excitement and agitation; it is also good for chorea (St. Vitus's dance), and all neuralgias.

Directions for use: 10-15 drops of the liquid extract should be taken in a little water three times daily.

BLACK HOREHOUND
(*Ballota nigra*)

'Black Horehound, good
For sheep or shepherd bitten by a mad-dog's venomed teeth.'

Faithful Shepherdess.

Also known as Madwort.

Description: Common in hedgerows and on waste land, it grows with leaves ovate, two at a joint opposite each other on leaf stalks, dented at the edges, dark green on top, paler underneath, with netted veins and slightly hairy. The stem grows from 1-4 ft. The flowers grow in whorls, the calyx being funnel-shaped, with short, spreading teeth and dilated at the mouth. The corolla is dark purple, the upper lip cleft, and is covered with small white hairs.

Part used: Leaves.

The botanical title comes from the Greek *ballo*, to reject, because of its disagreeable odour.

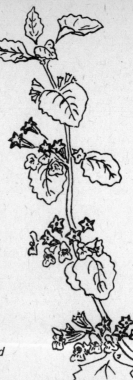

Black Horehound

Culpeper says, 'It is recommended as a remedy against hysteric, and hypochondriac affections'.

'This,' says Meyrick, 'is one of those neglected English herbs which are possessed of great virtues, though they are but little known, and still less regarded. It is superior to most things as a remedy in hysteria, and for low spirits'.

Richard Hool, an old herbalist, said, 'It should always be remembered that disease arises from obstruction, and until this obstruction is removed and any injury to the part is repaired, there is always a disturbance of the equilibrium of the blood circulation and the nerve force': black horsehound will restore this.

The herb soothes the nerves after coughing, and can be used with great benefit for nervous debility, loss of energy and in hysteria.

Instructions for use: Pour 1 pint of boiling water on to 1 oz of the dried leaves and when cold, strain.

A wineglassful should be taken three times a day.

BORAGE
(*Borago officinalis*)
'I Borage bring always courage.'
Greek proverb.

Also known as Burrage, Llanwenlys (Herb of Grace).
Description: This herb has been cultivated in England for generations, and it is also found in Europe. It usually grows on waste ground where the soil is sandy, and is about 12 inches high with an erect stem. The leaves are oval, greyish-green, about 3 inches long and 1½ inches broad, both leaves and stem are covered with stiff hairs. The flowers are bright blue.
Part used: The herb.

Most people know Borage as an ingredient in cider or claret cup and it is very good chopped up in salads.

Dr Fernie said that its reputed powers of invigoration could be medicinally substantiated for the juice contained 30 per cent nitrate of potash. The name is a corruption of *Cor-ago*, *cor* the heart and *ago*, I stimulate!

We read in the old books that countrymen used to place the leaves with cheese in sandwiches to provide sustaining nourishment.

Dioscorides said, 'Borage cheers the heart and helps drooping spirits'.

And in Gerard's *Herball* we find, 'Those of our time do use the floures in sallads, to exhilerate and make the minde glad. There be also many things made of them, used for the comfort of the heart, to drive away sorrow and increase the joy of the mind'.

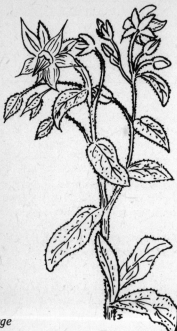

Borage

For centuries the flowers have had the reputation of curing melancholy and relieving depression of the nervous system and 'The sprigs of Borage,' wrote John Evelyn, 'are of known virtue to revive the hypochondriac and cheer the hard student'.

Another ancient author wrote:

'To enliven the sad with the joy of a joke,
Give them wine with some borage put in it to soak.'

So for depression and sorrow, remember Borage and drink it freely.

Directions for use: Make a tea by pouring 1 pint of boiling water on to 2 teaspoonsful of the dried herb. After five minutes or so it may be taken hot.

BUGLOSS
(*Echium vulgare*)

'. . . with bright blue eye
Your pains the Bugloss will repay,
And famed for driving care away
Dipped in a broader brighter blue,
Rough borage.'

Also known as Viper's Bugloss, Blueweed, Cat's tail.
Description: This herb grows in many places, in chalk
pits, on walls and in waste ground. It is from 1-2 ft high,
the leaves growing alternately up the stem, both covered
with prickly hairs. The leaves are small, long and pointed
at both ends. The flowers are bright blue, tubular,
funnel-shaped with four stamens protruding.
Part used: The herb.

Borage is characterized by its rough foliage with
bristly hairs. So rough and stiff are the almost prickly
hairs that Professor Martyn of Cambridge observed that
when bees come for honey they are apt to get their
wings torn. Incidentally bees love this plant as it is rich
in nectar.

It is known as Viper's Bugloss because the seed is
shaped like the head of a snake, and formerly it was
considered antidotal to the bite of a viper.

Culpeper says, 'It is a most gallant herb . . . the root
or seed is thought to be most effective to comfort the
heart and expel sadness or causeless melancholy'.

And from Dr Fernie: 'All herbs of the Borage order
(and this is one) are indifferently of force and virtue to
drive away sorrow and pensiveness of the mind; also to
comfort and strengthen the heart'.

This herb should not be forgotten in the treatment of
depression and sadness; also it relieves nervous headaches
and helps all nervous complaints.

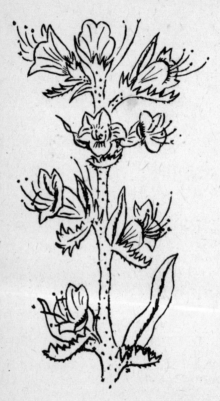

Bugloss

Directions for use: 1 pint of boiling water should be added to 1 oz of the herb and infused for twenty minutes. A cupful may be taken as and when required.

CATNEP
(*Nepita Cataria*)

'Lavender, Corn-rose, Pennyroyal sate,
And that which cats esteem delicate.'

Abraham Crawley.

Also known as Catmint or Nep.
Description: This herb grows in hedgerows and on waste ground and has become a common garden plant. It is 2-3 ft in height; the stems are square and at every junction there are two broad leaves, covered with down, nicked at the edges and aromatic. The flowers are purple-white and grow in tufts at the top of the branches and lower down the stems.

Gerard says, 'the whole plant is soft and covered with a white down. All parts have a pungent smell'.
Part used: The herb.

Gerard called it Herba Cattaria, 'because cats are very much delighted herewith; for the smell of it is so pleasant unto them that they rub themselves upon it and wallow and tumble in it, and also feed on the branches and leaves very greedily'.

Rats object to this plant, so much so that if grown thickly they will not go through, however hungry they may be.

Culpeper said, 'It is a good medicine allaying hysteria and soothing to the nervous system, and is so safe it can have no harmful effects'.

Catnep is very valuable to relieve pain after eating when the *cause* is either anaemia or nervous debility. It is soothing to the nervous system, especially in hysterical people, relaxing and helpful in all cases of nervousness.

Hoffman said, 'The root of catmint, if chewed, will make the most gentle person fierce and quarrelsome'. And there is a legend about a certain hangman who

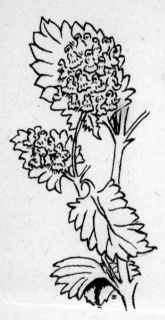

Catnap

could never find the courage for his gruesome task until he had masticated some of the aromatic root. This proves that catnep will tone up the nervous system and supply more energy.

Directions for use: An infusion is made by pouring a pint of boiling water on to 1 oz of the herb; it will make a great difference if this is covered as soon as the water has been added, instead of allowing it to be exposed to the air. It can be sweetened with honey if desired. Drink hot as a tea.

CHAMOMILE
(*Anthemis nobilis*)

'The camomile shall teach patience
Which riseth best when trodden most upon.'

(From an early seventeenth century play.)

Also known as Roman chamomile, Grand Apple, Whig
Plant.

Description: This herb is found in England but more
plentifully in Belgium and France. The true chamomile
grows prostrate and produces one flower on a stem
which resembles the daisy, with a convex yellow disc,
whilst its leaves are divided into hair-like segments.

Part used: The flowers and herb.

In some parts of England chamomile grows wild, but
the old-fashioned gardens were imperfect without a bed
of these flowers, which were employed during the winter
for making into tea for various complaints.

It was used in early days to make a fragrant 'lawn' for
as Falstaff said to Henry, Prince of Wales, soon to
become King Henry V: 'Harry, I do not only marvel
where thou spendest thy time, but also how thou art
accompanied; for though the camomile, the more it is
trodden the faster it grows, yet youth, the more it is
wasted the sooner it wears'.

Dr Fernie says, 'This flower was well known to the
Greeks who thought it had an odour like that of apples
and therefore named it "Earth Apple" from two of their
words, *Kamai* meaning on the ground, and *melon*, an
apple. The Spaniards call it *Manzanilla* from a little
apple, and gave the name to one of their lightest sherries
flavoured with this plant'.

In Elizabethan times, before tobacco was brought to
England, the leaves were dried and smoked, and the
aroma helped sleeplessness.

The flowers of chamomile have a strong aromatic smell and a peculiar bitter taste. When distilled with water they give off a small quantity of a very useful essential oil, which is blue in colour. Medicinally this oil lowers nervous excitement reflected from an organ in the body which is not working efficiently, such as nervous colic from the bowels.

Chamomile tea is drunk in many parts of the world regularly. It is a cleansing tonic and soothing to the nerves, and nervous complaints of women. This tea would be good taken during the time of the menopause.

For nervous headache a combination of chamomile and peppermint is excellent.

Directions for use: 2-4 drops of the oil may be taken as a dose on sugar or in milk.

A tea is made by pouring boiling water on to a teaspoonful of flowers for each person in a teapot (to

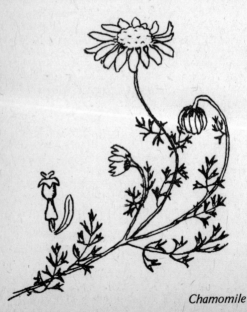

Chamomile

prevent the steam escaping as this impairs its properties), and this should stand for at least ten minutes before being poured off. It should be taken before or after meals. Lemon or orange peel may be added for flavouring.

An infusion of chamomile and peppermint should be made by pouring 1 quart of boiling water on to ½ oz of each herb mixed together; when cold this should be strained and taken freely.

HERB BENNET
(*Geum urbanum*)

'Nor herb nor flow'ret glistened there
But was carved in the cloister arches as fair.'

Also known as Avens, Holy Herb, Colewort, Way Bennet and Wild Rye.

Description: It grows wild in the shade and under hedges in Great Britain and Europe. This herb has many long rough dark green leaves rising from the root. There are many hairy stalks about 2 ft high branching with trefoiled leaves at every joint. On the top of the branches are small, pale yellow flowers, consisting of five leaves, in the middle of which is a small green web which, when the flower has fallen, grows to be round, being made of many long greenish-purple seeds which will stick to clothing. The root consists of many brownish strings smelling rather like cloves.

Part used: The herb and root.

Herb Bennet is said to be a corruption of *Herba benedicta*, which means 'blessed herb' and is applied to this little plant because, says an old tradition, where the root is in the house, the devil can do nothing and flies from it; so it is blessed above all other herbs.

Geum is from the Greek *Geuo* — 'to yield an agreeable fragrance' — which is true of the roots.

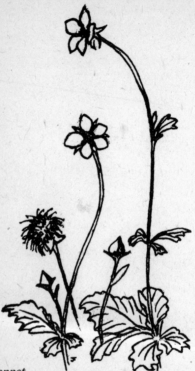

Herb Bennet

Dr Fernie tells us that 'It's graceful trefoiled leaf and the fine golden petals of it's flowers, symbolizing the five wounds of Christ, were sculptured by the monks in the thirteenth century on their church architecture'.

This herb restores strength to the economy, and is a good tonic in general debility, which must include the nervous system.

Directions for use: ½ pint of boiling water should be poured on to 3 teaspoonsful of the dried or fresh herb.

This should be strained after ten minutes and a wineglassful taken three times daily. This should be taken over a long period.

HOLY THISTLE
(*Carduus benedictus*)

'Get you some of this distilled Carduus benedictus and lay it on your heart; it is the only thing for a qualm. I mean plain Holy Thistle.'

Shakespeare

Also known as Blessed Thistle, Milk Thistle, Spotted Thistle.

Description: Leaves greyish green, thin and brittle, irregularly toothed ending at the spine; the flowers grow on top of the stalk and are about 1 inch long and 1¾ inches broad and yellow in colour.

Part used: The Herb.

Carduus or Cadinal refers to the spring leaves and benedictus gives it the name of Holy.

An old writer says of this plant, 'It is called Carduus benedictus, or Blessed Thistle or Holy Thistle; I suppose the name was put upon it by some that had little holiness in themselves. It is an herb of Mars and under the sign of Aries. It helpeth swimmings and giddiness of the head, or the disease called Vertigo, because Aries is in the house of Mars. It strengthens the attractive faculty in man and clarifies the blood because the one is ruled by Mars'.

William Coles tells us in his *Knowledge of Plants* that if the down flies off coltsfoot, dandelion or thistles when there is no wind, it is a certain sign of rain.

We are told that it was first cultivated by Gerard in 1597 and has been used for many years as a 'simple'.

This herb helps to purify and circulate the blood and so it is excellent in so many ways, and it helps to soothe

the nerves and brain and strengthen the memory.

Dioscorides said of this thistle, 'The root if borne about one, doth expel melancholy and remove all diseases connected therewith'.

It should be remembered, therefore, in cases of depression and the various symptoms which spring from it.

Directions for use: 2 oz of the dried plant should be

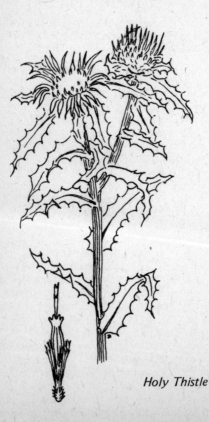

Holy Thistle

simmered in a quart of water for two hours. The dose is
a wineglassful and this is best taken on going to bed.

HOPS
(*Humulus lupulus*)

'In the reign of Henry VI a person was proceeded
against for putting into beer "an unwholesome
weed called an hopp".'
From *Potters New Cyclopaedia.*

Description: Hops grow in hedgerows and woodlands
throughout England and, of course, they are cultivated
— mostly in Kent — for brewing. The stems are long,
climbing; the leafy female strobile (flower) consists of
membranous scales which are yellowish-green and oval.
Part used: Flowers (strobiles).

The word hop comes from the Anglo-Saxon *hoppan*,
to climb.

Hops were first brought to England in 1524 when
they were used for brewing. Before then, ale was made
from malt and clarified by ground ivy (ale-hoof).

It is said that hops will produce sleep when nothing
else will and 'a pillow, pulvinar humuli, stuffed with
newly dried hops' says Dr Fernie, 'was successfully
prescribed by Dr Willis for George III, when sedative
medicines had failed to give him sleep'.

Directions for use: A tablespoonful of the dried flowers
should be simmered in a pint of water for ten minutes.
When cool it should be strained and ½ pint taken night
and morning. For facial neuralgia a hot fomentation
should be made by pouring sufficient boiling water on to
a handful of the flowers to make them moist and hot,
then the remaining water should be squeezed out, and
the flowers placed between two layers of linen and
applied to the affected part. This can be repeated as

often as is necessary. Care should be taken not to burn
the skin.

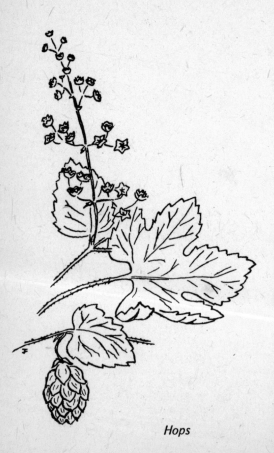

Hops

LADY'S SLIPPER
(*Cypripedum pubescens*)

'Oh who can tell
The hidden power of herbs and might of magick
spell.'   *Spenser.*

Also known as Lady's shoe, Nerve-root, Noah's Ark,
Yellow Lady's Slipper.

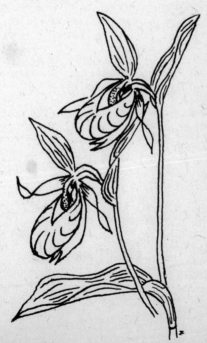

Lady's Slipper

Description: This is one of the rarest and most beautiful of the British wild flowers; it is now almost extinct except in Yorkshire and Durham. It has a creeping root from which a downy stalk rises to about 12 inches. The leaves are broad, pale green and heavily ribbed and there are three or four on each stem. At the top of the stem there is one flower with reddish, sometimes twisted sepals, and a large inflated yellow lip, which attracts the bees. The flowers are large and showy and when newly open they have a very soft sweet perfume.

Part used: The root.

This herb is used for healing and it has great relaxing properties, and so quietens the nerves. Its influence is slow but is centred entirely on the nervous system. It is excellent as a general nerve tonic and can be prescribed for most nervous troubles including irritability and hysteria.

Dr England of America recommended the mixture of scullcap, lady's slipper and capsicum for nervous complaints adding 'the capsicum helps the influence of the other ingredients'.

Directions for use: 1 teaspoonful of the powdered root should be taken in sweetened water as a dose.

The mixture should be obtained from a medical herbalist.

LIME FLOWERS
(*Tilia europoso*)

'To the lime flower
    We see you not; but we scarce know why
    We are glad when the air you have breathed goes by
    Hail blossoms green 'mid the limes unseen
    That charm the bees to your honey's screen
    We see you not . . .'
                Sir Aubrey de Vere.

Also known as Linnflowers or Linden flowers.

Description: A large tree indigenous to Britain and to most parts of Europe. It has smooth dark brown bark with spreading branches round in a regular manner; the leaves are heart-shaped with serrated edges; and from them grow the stalks upon which are a cluster of pendulous yellowish white flowers, with stamens equalling the number of petals. The flowers are powerfully scented but are hardly seen as they are hidden by the leaves which are almost the same colour.

Part used: The flowers.

In the old herbals the tree is called Lyne or Line, Tillet, Till tree and Tilia, the latter probably derived from ptilon, a feather because of the feathery appearance of the floral leaves.

Pliny tells us that the Romans used to boil the inner bark of the linden tree with meat that was too salt, and that in his day chaplets were made from the bark.

The linden or lime tree was the ancient emblem of Germanic countries, and to this day lime trees are to be found in villages throughout Germany, many of them having been planted centuries ago.

The sweet smelling and highly fragrant flowers blossom in June and are very popular with bees as they contain so much nectar.

'The wood of the lime tree is preferred before any other for masterly carving. Grinling Gibbons executed his best and most noted work in this material; and the finely cut details still remain sharp, delicate and beautiful', so Dr Fernie tells us.

Lime flower tea (tilleuil) is widely known in France as an after dinner drink as it soothes the nerves and helps to induce sleep. It is an excellent remedy for nervous and catarrhal symptoms following a cold. Restless people benefit from lime flowers and it is very good for hysteria.

Lime flowers are beneficial when used in a warm bath for nervous irritability.

Directions for use: A tea is made by pouring boiling water on to a teaspoonful of flowers for each person in a teapot, and after standing for ten minutes it should be

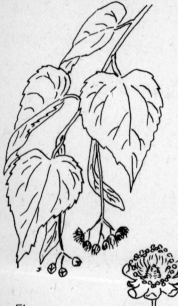

Lime Flowers

taken hot as often as needed. For a full bath about 10 oz of lime flowers made into an infusion and allowed to stand for about ten minutes, should be strained and added to the bath water.

MARJORAM
(*Origanum vulgare*)

'The pleasant way as up the hills you climb
Is strewed o're with marjoram and thyme
Which grows unset.'

George Withers.

Also known as Candy.

Description: It grows on dry, hilly pastures and banks; it is about 12 inches tall and has broad ovate leaves, short stalked and covered with down. The flowers grow in clusters on the top of each stem, they are rosy-red.

Part used: The herb.

This herb has a sweet aromatic scent which is very refreshing. In olden times 'sweet waters' were made from the leaves and sprinkled in the rooms of large houses.

Gerard says, 'The leaves boiled in water, and the decoction drunke, easeth such as are given to overmuch sighing'.

Marjoram stimulates the appetite and probably this is why it is added to so many dishes in cooking.

The crushed dried leaves were used as snuff.

It is a very good tonic and will relieve a nervous headache. It is excellent for the whole nervous system and indigestion.

Directions for use: Make a tea by putting 2 teaspoonsful of the dried herb into a 1½ pint teapot and fill with boiling water. Leave for at least 5 minutes before drinking. It may be sweetened with honey if desired.

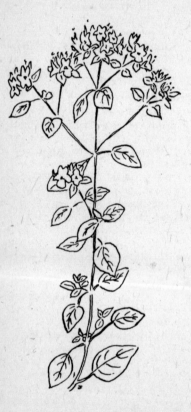

Marjoram

MISTLETOE
(*Viscum album*)

'Now with bright holly all the Temples strow
With laurel, green and sacred Mistletoe.'

Gay.

Also known as Birdlime Mistletoe, European Mistletoe.
Culpeper spells it 'Messelto'.

Description: It has a woody stem growing out of the tree
from which it gets its nourishment, with many branches
interlaced, covered with a yellow-green bark. The leaves
grow opposite, they are leathery and long. The small
yellow flowers grow at the joints of the branches,
subsequently producing small round white translucent
berries. It is evergreen.

Part used: The leaves and dried young twigs.

The thrush devours the berries and soils or 'missels'
his feet with the viscid seeds and thus conveys them
from tree to tree; this is how he gets the name of 'Missel
thrush'.

This herb was held in great veneration by the druids
who gathered it with a golden sickle after a vision
directing them to cut it.

Coles tells us that if people hang mistletoe about their
necks the witches can have no power against them!

The celebrated mistletoe bough was famous 'for
further and more noble purposes than barely to feed
thrushes, or to be hung up superstitiously in houses to
drive away evil spirits', says Sir J. Colbach, by which we
learn that great faith was put in this mystic plant.

We are told that the farmers in Worcestershire used to
take their bough of mistletoe and give it to the cow who
calved first after New Year's Day, as this was supposed
to avert ill-luck from the whole dairy.

It is used in many homes today at Christmas time but

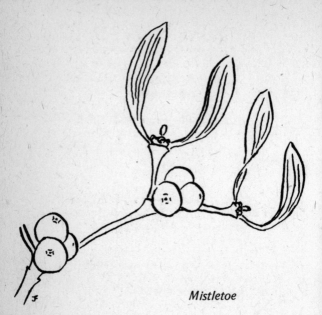

Mistletoe

is banned in most churches as a symbol of paganism.

A French author of many years ago says, 'Mistletoe may be taken in decoction against all sorts of nervous maladies . . . it gives tone to the nerves if taken in the morning and on going to bed and re-establishes the circulation of the blood'.

It is in general use as a nerve tonic, and it will clear up many complaints arising from a weakened and dis-ordered state of the nervous system, such as nervous debility, hysteria, neuralgia, etc.

It is claimed to be very effective in the cure of chorea or St. Vitus's dance.

A useful prescription for all nervous complaints is mistletoe, valerian and vervain.

Directions for use: 1 oz of the young leaves should be boiled in 1 pint of water for about ten minutes; this should then be strained and a wineglassful taken three or four times daily. For the combination mix together ½ oz each of mistletoe, valerian root and vervain; boil in 1½ pints of water for ten minutes. When cool it should be strained and a small wineglassful taken two or three times daily.

MOTHERWORT
(*Leonurus cardiaca*)

' . . . Even in the green herb have I given
you all things.'
Genesis 9:3.

Also known as Lion's Ear, Lion's Tail.
Description: This herb grows wild in Britain and commonly in gardens. The stem is square, growing to 3 ft and spreading into many branches; the lower leaves are five-lobed and the upper three-lobed, two leaves grow at every joint. The flowers grow in dense whorls in the axils of the upper leaves, white or pink, purple spotted.
Part used: The herb.
   Culpeper says, 'There is no better herb to take melancholy vapours from the heart, and strengthen it'.
   Motherwort is very useful in nervous complaints, especially hysteria and fainting. It is most helpful in complaints of women when there is weakness with hysteria; it is an excellent tonic for the generative organs and helps to allay irritability.
Directions for use: An infusion is made by pouring 1 pint of boiling water on to 1 oz of the dried herb. When cold a wineglassful should be taken three times daily.

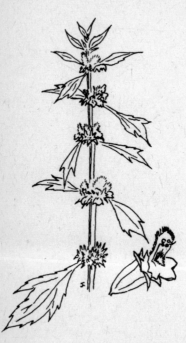

Motherwort

OATS
(*Avena Sativa*)

'Cuckoo Oats and Woodcock Hay
Makes a farmer run away.'

Also known as Groats.
Description: Fields of oats are distinguished from corn
as at the top of the main stem there are spikes of 'ears'
hanging on slender pedicels.
Part used: The seed.

From the rhyme we understand that if the spring is so
backward that the oats cannot be sown till the cuckoo is
heard, or the autumn is so wet that the hay cannot be
gathered till the woodcocks come over, the farmer is
sure to suffer great loss!

From earliest times, oats have been the staple food
for the horse, and wherever this animal was introduced,
oats were grown for his use.

'Physicians formerly recommended a diet drink made
from oats about which Hoffman wrote a treatise at the
end of the seventeenth century; and Johannis de
St Catherine, who introduced the drink, lived by its use
to 100 years free from any disease', says Dr Fernie.

Porridge made from oats as a breakfast food has very
largely declined in popularity and has been replaced by
modern packet food such as corn-flakes, etc. It is felt,
however, that this is a retrograde step as the Scots had
the reputation of being very strong and fit, and their
breakfast for generations, consisted of oatmeal porridge.
In the border forays of centuries ago all the provisions
which the Scots carried was a bag of oatmeal.

Avena Sativa is especially valuable in cases of over-
tired nerves, and in sleeplessness from nervous exhaustion. It is an excellent nerve tonic; it restores nervous
prostration and removes depression.

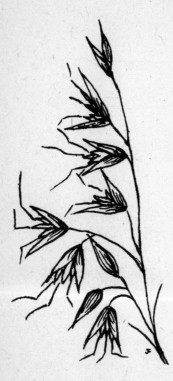

Oats

Directions for use: 10-20 drops of the fluid extract should be taken in a little water three times daily after meals.

PASSION FLOWER
(*Passiflora incarnata*)

'The Passion Flower long has blow'd
To betoken us signs of the Holy Rood.'

Also known as Maypops.

Description: It is a tropical plant and is grown in
England in greenhouses. It climbs and has three-lobed
oval heart-shaped leaves. The flowers grow singly on

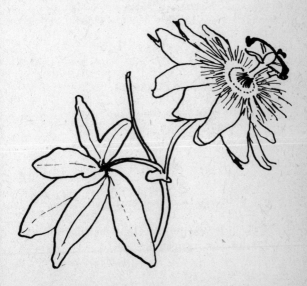

Passion Flower

each stem and are white with purple centres and are very beautiful. In its native country branches of the passion flower often climb to the tops of the highest trees where they sustain themselves by means of tendrils.

Part used: Plant and leaves.

This flower is traditionally associated with the Crucifixion and we are told that the Spanish friars in America first called it 'flower of the Passion'.

This herb is widely used as a sedative and is excellent for quieting the nerves and nervous system. It can be taken during the daytime without any fear of the brain being dulled.

It is especially helpful in calming nervous restlessness during the menopause, which can be such a difficult time for many women. It soothes neuralgic pains and irritations and assists the nervous system to recover during convalescence.

Nervous headaches and hysteria both respond to this herbal remedy.

Directions for use: It is best to purchase the liquid extract of this herb and the dose is 10-20 drops in water three times daily.

Tablets also may be purchased from some health food stores and the dose is given on the bottle.

ROSEMARY
(*Rosmarinus officinalis*)

'There's Rosemary, thats for remembrance,
Pray you love, remember me.'

Shakespeare.

Also known as Romero.

Description: It is a common plant in Britain and was cultivated here prior to the Norman conquest. The stem is rather woody, square, the leaves are narrow and short, dark green above and silver below, hairy; the flowers are

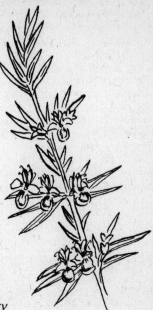

Rosemary

blue-lilac, two lipped with only two stamens. It is very aromatic.
Part used: The herb.

An ancient writer explains the name by saying that Rosemary is the plant that grows by the sea (*mare*) from which *marinus* is derived. Another writer says that rose, the first part of the name is from *ros*, (dew) as the plant is often seen glittering with dew on the shores of the sea.

In a very old book the virtues of Rosemary are discussed thus: 'The flowers are preferred to the leaves; they are good against rheumatism, nervous disposition, general debility and especially weakness of vision, melancholy, weak circulation and cramp'.

Sir Thomas More says, 'I lett it run alle over my

garden walls, not onlie because my bees love it, but because 'tis the herb sacred to remembrance, and therefore friendship; whence a sprig of it hath a dum language that maketh it the chosen emblem of our funeral wakes and in our buriall grounds'.

In the French flower language this herb is supposed to represent the power of re-kindling lost energy and the ancients said that it refreshed the memory and comforted the brain.

Rosemary tea will soon relieve hysterical depression and it is very good for headaches caused by nervousness; it also stimulates the nervous system.

Directions for use: Put 1 teaspoonful of the dried herb in a 1½ pint teapot, fill with boiling water and let it stand for at least five minutes. Drink as a tea.

SAGE
(*Salvia officinalis*)

'Sage helps the nerves, and by its powerful might
Palsey is cured and fever put to flight.'

An old French rhyme.

Also known as Garden sage.
Description: Growing about 2 ft tall it has hairy stems with long rough leaves, greyish-green, which release an aromatic smell when handled. The flowers are brilliant blue. It is found on grassy downlands and where the soil is calcareous, and it now grows in many herb and country gardens.
Part used: The leaves.

This is a very well known herb growing in many gardens in England and it is a pity that relatively few people know more about its merits than as an ingredient in 'sage and onion stuffing' which accompanies roast pork or duck!

Sage is known in many other countries and wherever

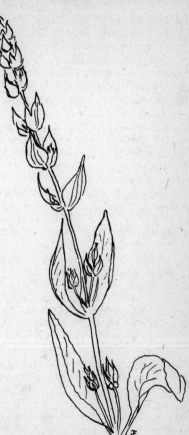

Sage

it grows it is used domestically.

It was given pride of place over other garden plants by the ancients, and Walafrid Strabo wrote in the ninth century, 'Amongst my herbs, sage holds place of honour; of good scent it is and full of virtue for many ills'.

There is an old saying, 'Why should a man die whilst sage grows in his garden?' and in some parts of England the following advice is given, but whether it is still carried out it is difficult to say!

> 'He that would live for aye
> Must eat sage in May.'

In one county in England it was maintained that the wife rules where sage grows vigorously and also that the plant would thrive or decline as the master's business prospered or failed!

Salvia is derived from the Latin *Salvere* which means 'to save' and this herb was regarded highly by Gerard who says, 'Sage is singular good for the head and brain; it quickeneth the senses and memory, strengtheneth the sinuses; restoreth health to those that hath the palsey, and takes away shaky trembling of the members'.

It is said that this herb mitigates grief, mental and bodily.

Those who suffer from any nervous complaints will benefit from drinking sage tea which is very pleasant, and incidentally was one of the main drinks in this country before Indian and China teas were imported. It is excellent for nerve exhaustion.

The Chinese are as fond of sage as we are of their tea, and they cannot understand why we purchase so much China tea when we grow sage in this country, which they consider far superior with all its healing properties.

It was thought that sage, if used in the making of cheese would improve its flavour, and sage cheese can be purchased occasionally to this day — the green colour of the herb running through the yellow makes quite an attractive variation.

Directions for use: To make sage tea pour 1 pint of boiling water on to 2 teaspoonsful of the dried leaves and let it stand for six minutes — a cup should be taken three times daily.

SCULLCAP
(*Scutellaria lateriflora*)

'He causeth the grass to grow for the cattle,
and herb for the service of man.'

Psalms 104:14

Also known as Hood Wort, Helmet Flower, Madweed,
and Quaker Bonnet.

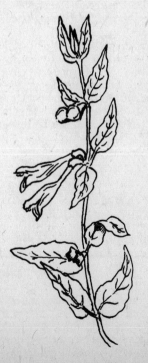

Scullcap

Description: This herb has square stems, leaves grow opposite and are heart shaped but pointed at both ends. The flowers are blue with helmet-shaped upper lip.
Part used: The herb.

This herb gets its name from the Latin *scutella*, 'a little cap', which the calyx resembles.

Scullcap does much to restore any disorders of the nervous system and is especially helpful in nervous twitching. It is very quieting and soothing to the nerves of people who are easily excited and it also helps those who are confused in their minds. It is useful in neuralgia and soothes a person to sleep if suffering from an exhausted brain.

A valuable recipe for nervous headaches, restlessness, hysteria and other nervous symptoms is equal parts of scullcap and valerian.

Directions for use: An infusion of 1 pint of boiling water should be added to 1 oz of the herb and strained when cool. A wineglassful should be taken three or four times daily. Also ½ oz of scullcap powder and ½ oz valerian powder should be well mixed and 1 teaspoonful stirred into a cupful of boiling water and when cooled, this should be taken as one dose. To be repeated two or three times daily.

VALERIAN
(*Valeriana officinalis*)

'They that will have their heale
Must put Setwall in their keale.'

An old saying.

Also known as Great Wild Valerian, Vandal root, Setwall, Heal-all and Capon's tail, the latter from its spreading flowers. Valerian is from *valere*, to be well.
Description: This herb grows in wet meadows, banks of streams, copses, etc. The stem is erect, downy and about

2 ft high. The bottom leaves are broad and long but those that are higher on the stem are deeply divided along each side, some to the middle rib. Small clusters of pink flowers grow on stalks from the main stem. The

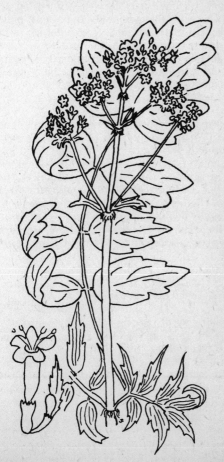

Valerian

root has a very disagreeable odour. The root stock is short, thick and greyish with numerous short, lateral branches and rootlets.

Part used: The root.

Valerian is a benedicta or Blessed herb, being dedicated to the Virgin Mary as a preservative against poison.

The spikenard of the ancients is now known to be a member of the valerian family.

This plant is often described as having mystical properties and the Greeks employed one kind of valerian for hanging up at doors and windows as a charm.

Cats are fascinated by the roots and become almost intoxicated if they nibble at them.

It is known in the North of England as Setwall and, says Gerard, 'No broths, pottage, or physical meats be worth anything if Setwall be not there.' Preparations of this herb relieve nervous headaches associated with flatulence in a person of nervous temperament. It is excellent for nervous exhaustion brought on by emotional excitement. Valerian gives great comfort in cases of nervous debility and is very useful in times of strain and tiredness. It has general calming effects and is, in fact, a welcome tranquillizer without having any side effects.

A combination of valerian, scullcap, vervain and mistletoe is most helpful in restlessness, insomnia, neuralgia and general nervous debility.

Directions for use: This root should never be boiled. 1 pint of boiling water may be poured on to 1 oz of the powdered root and allowed to cool, and a small wineglassful taken three times daily. A more effective preparation is as follows: 1 teaspoonful of the powdered root should be soaked in a cup of cold water for 12 hours: this should be strained and taken one hour before retiring. The other prescription is: take ½ oz each of scullcap, vervain, mistletoe and valerian root and boil in 3 pints of water down to a quart; when cold a wineglassful should be taken four times daily. (This is from a very old herbal and the boiling with other herbs seems to be effective.)

Valerian should not be taken for too long periods; after a course of three or four weeks a break of a fortnight is advisable; then it can be repeated as and when necessary.

VERVAIN
(*Verbena officinalis*)

'Trefoil, Vervain, John's Wort, Dill,
Hinder witches of their will.'

Also known as American Vervain, Wild Hyssop, Blue Vervain, Simpler's Joy, Traveller's Joy, Pigeon's Grass, Holy Herb, Juno's tears and Herb of Grace. The leaf is called Frog's Foot!
Description: Culpeper states, 'It grows generally throughout the land in divers places of the hedges and waysides and other waste ground'. Vervain is a slender plant growing to a height of 1-2 ft with broad leaves next to the ground, deeply gashed about the edges, and stalks branching with small flowers, two lipped and of pinkish blue, on each sprig. It was probably cultivated in herb gardens. When rubbed, the odour is slightly aromatic.
Part used: The herb.

Vervain is derived from an old Celtic word meaning 'to drive away'.

The Druids gathered verbena with as much reverence as they paid to mistletoe. It is one of the herbs which could be used by, or against witches!

The heads of the Roman priests were sometimes garlanded with vervain, which they called the sacred or magic herb.

The plant was dedicated to Isis, the Goddess of Birth.

Pliny wrote, 'They report that if the dining chamber be sprinkled with water in which the herb verbena has been steeped, the guests will be the merrier'.

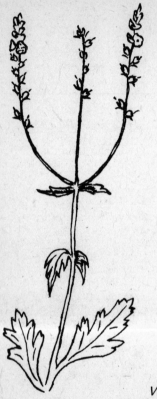

Vervain

Vervain grew on Calvary and Gerard says, 'The devil did reveal it as a secret and divine medicine'.

This is a most useful herb for nervousness, sleeplessness and nervous headache. It will tone up the whole nervous system, thus acting as a general nerve tonic. It helps to relieve nervous exhaustion and acts as a sedative.

Directions for use: A pint of boiling water should be

added to 1 oz of the herb; after straining, a wineglassful should be taken three times daily. This may be sweetened with a little honey if desired.

WOOD BETONY
(*Betonica officinalis*)

'. . . and the fruit thereof shall be for meat,
and the leaf thereof for medicine.'

Ezekiel 47:12

Also known as Bishopwort, Lousewort.
Description: This plant grows wild chiefly in shady woods and meadows. It is quite small, having many leaves rising from the root which are rather broad and rounded at the ends and dented at margins; the central stem of about 1 ft high has smaller leaves and at the top are several spiked heads of flowers rather like lavender but thicker and shorter, of purple or reddish colour with white spots. The stem is square, slender and hairy.
Part used: The leaves.

Wood Betony is a wonderful herb with many uses, one being a dark yellow dye for wool.

An old author tells us that 'the wort that one names betonicum is produced in meadows and on clean soils; it is good for man's soul and for his body; it shields him against monstrous nocturnal visitors and against visions and dreams'. Pliny says it was first named 'Vettonica' in honour of the Vettones, a people of Spain.

Country people used to call this plant 'Bitny'. The name 'betonica' is from the Celtic *ben* meaning head and *tonic* meaning good, thus describing this herb as being very good for all pains in the head and face; it is also used for neuralgia and all nervous ailments.

Betony used to be very highly thought of by people of many countries and there is an old Italian proverb which says, 'sell your coat and buy betony' and in more

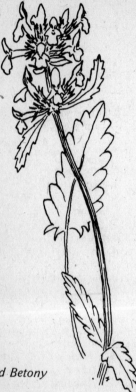

Wood Betony

recent times when speaking of somebody they respect, they say, 'He has as many virtues as betony'.

Antonius Musa, chief physician to the Emperor Augustus, wrote a book entirely on the virtues of this herb.

Culpeper wrote, 'This is a precious herb well worth

keeping in your home. It is so wholesome it cannot be misused'.

For a languid nervous headache betony tea is most beneficial; and a combination of betony, scullcap and rosemary is excellent for neuralgia and as a nerve tonic. *Directions for use:* Betony tea is made by simmering 2 oz of the dried herb in a quart of water until 1½ pints remain. A wineglassful should be taken three times daily.

For the other prescription, add one quart of boiling water to 1 oz wood betony, ½ oz scullcap and ½ oz rosemary — let it steep for 20 minutes, strain and a wineglassful should be taken three or four times daily.

HONEY
(*Mel.*)

'. . . they traded in thy market wheat of
Minnith, and Pen-nag and honey, and oil
and balm.'

Ezekiel 27:17

Honey is essentially of flower and herb origin; the nectar from which the bees produce it is obtained from a wide variety of plants, and as honey has curative properties it is included in this work.

The name honey is derived from a Hebrew word *ghoneg* which means literally 'delight'.

Honey dates from the oldest times of the known world and in the Bible we read that the land of Canaan, where Abraham dwelt, was flowing with milk and honey. In the Mosaic law there were statutes regulating the ownership of bees.

Pliny, in one of his books on Natural History devotes many chapters to honey 'which bees collect from sweet juices of flowers so beneficial to health'. He tells us of Romilius Pollio, who enjoyed marvellous health and vitality when over one hundred years old. He was presented to Emperor Augustus, who asked what was the secret of his wondrous longevity and Pollio answered, 'The eating of honey and anointing outside with oil'.

Honey cakes in those days were made for feasts with meal, honey and oil.

Honey was not only used as a food then, but also in surgery as its antiseptic and healing properties were widely known. It was applied to ulcerations of the skin and was used as an ointment or plaster for boils, burns and wounds, and sometimes it was mixed with other ingredients. Another use was to put a drop into inflamed eyes, for which it was, and still is, a most effective remedy.

A very popular drink in Roman times was made of fruit with added honey, and before hops were used in the brewing of beers, honey was the basis of mead, the drink of olden times. Queen Elizabeth was very fond of mead and had it made regularly according to her own recipe, which included the leaves of sweet briar, rosemary, cloves and mace. Recently there has been a revival of interest in mead and it is now available in small quantities.

It would be very beneficial if we were to copy our forefathers of old and use honey as they did. However in the scope of this book its curative properties must be discussed in relation to nervous conditions. Honey can play an important role in the treatment of all nervous disorders as it helps to build up a strong nervous system.

In the building of a healthy body it is necessary to take foods and drinks that feed every part of the economy, and honey is speedily absorbed into the blood stream without placing strain on the digestion.

It consists of two natural sugars, enzymes and vitamins, and it supplies nourishment, heat and energy. On the other hand, white sugar is a habit forming stimulant which supplies heat and energy but no nourishment because all the nutritive elements are destroyed in the manufacture and refining processes; it is also acid forming.

Honey is superior to the brown sugars, although in present day diets it is difficult to dispense entirely with products containing sugar, but it should be born in mind that where possible sugar should be replaced with honey and when sugar must be taken then Barbados or Demerara are better than white.

One of the reasons why emphasis is on the use of honey in preference to sugar is that in highly concentrated form, sugars are powerful stimulants, they oxidize in the human stomach upon contact with oxygen, producing strain upon the digestive system which causes vital organs to work harder. This, in turn, has an effect on the nervous system which needs gentle feeding rather than violent stimulation. It cannot be denied that sugar can produce a great stimulation — a sense of exhilatation — a lift — but it should be remembered that there *must* be a swing of the pendulum, and this *lift* will be followed by depression. One could be led into a false sense of well-being by constantly taking sugar in order to continue the 'lift' and thus a habit is formed.

Honey provides the same sense of well-being but, being a natural unrefined product, it does not have any ill-effects.

When overtired, after hard work and strain, a spoonful of honey in warm water will help to overcome the fatigue very rapidly.

Honey helps to soothe the nerves and in hot milk last thing at night promotes sound sleep.

There is a great variety of honey available today but it is advisable to ascertain, when purchasing, that the product is pure unadulterated honey.

Unfortunately, there are a very few people who cannot tolerate honey and they should cut to the minimum their intake of white sugar, and substitute Barbados, but even then, the least possible quantity should be taken.

SUPPLEMENTARY ADVICE

In dealing with nervous troubles, it is necessary to realize that nerves need food to nourish them as they are part of the whole economy.

The diet therefore, should be studied, and foods which help to maintain the nervous system should be taken freely.

Most nervously distraught people are found to be deficient in either trace elements, (such as copper, cobalt, iron or manganese); or minerals (phosphorus and potassium). Others are seriously lacking in vitamins, especially B6 which is found abundantly in wheatgerm oil, egg yolk, herrings, whole wheat bread and fresh leafy vegetables.

Among the foods containing the trace elements copper, cobalt, iron and manganese, the most important are:

Copper: Brewer's yeast, lobster, wheat, bananas, brazil nuts, crayfish, avocado pears, spinach, liver, All-bran, mackerel, mushrooms, dried peas, oats, prunes, eggs, oysters.

Cobalt: Turnip greens, lettuce, spinach, beet tops, cabbage, figs, pears, onions, green peas, carrots, tomatoes, Swiss chard, walnuts, apricots.

Iron: Kidney, liver, egg-yolk, bran, dried peaches, molasses, dried peas, figs, mutton, oatmeal, raisins, beef, green vegetables, eggs, dried fruits, whole cereals, cabbage, white fish, apples.

Manganese: Oatmeal, whole wheat flour, lettuce, rice (brown), spinach, beetroot, kale, prunes, citrus fruits, nuts, egg yolk. And among the foods containing the trace elements are:

Phosphorus: Cheddar cheese and dried milk, eggs, whole cereals, meat, fish and poultry, dried fruits, fresh fruits, nuts and vegetables.

Potassium: Celery, apples, potatoes in their jackets,

peas, wholewheat, veal, almonds, cottage cheese, lamb, lean beef, watercress, lentils, raisins, figs and grapes.

Only 100 per cent. wholemeal bread should be eaten as it includes the germ of the wheat which is an important vitamin. (If too much roughage cannot be tolerated for reasons of ulceration, etc., it is possible to obtain a much finer flour of 81 per cent. extraction which is the next best thing.

Honey should be taken daily and it ought to replace white sugar wherever possible. It is important to study the section on honey earlier in this book.

Potatoes should always be well scrubbed and baked in their jackets and the whole eaten, as valuable minerals are present just under the skin. The practice of peeling potatoes robs the food of much of its value.

Vegetables should be cooked conservatively in saucepans of enamel or stainless steel. *Aluminium should always be avoided.* This applies also when boiling herbs, or the water to pour on a tea. The vegetables should be placed in the saucepan with very little water and a tightly fitting lid, and simmered gently until tender; over-cooking should be avoided as the vegetables then become mushy.

Always remember that raw vegetables and fruit are superior to those that have been cooked, as they have not been robbed of any of their vitamins or mineral content.

A fresh salad should be taken every day including, when in season, watercress, mustard and cress, lettuce, grated raw cabbage and carrot, tomatoes, peppers, raw mushrooms, and cucumber if it can be digested. Grated sprouts are delicious when in season and so is grated raw beetroot in addition to the usual cooked variety.

Fresh fruits, with or without yogurt, nuts and raisins should replace puddings and pies.

Cheese, eggs, fish, meat and poultry should all be taken in moderation.

From the above a good, wholesome mixed diet, containing protein, carbohydrates, vitamins and minerals and a small amount of starch can be prepared.

Early morning and late evening hot drinks (tea, coffee and cocoa) should be replaced by herbal teas discussed under the herbs concerned. The drinking of tea and coffee should be cut to the minimum and then only taken if it is very weak.

Fresh air and exercise are of the utmost importance. A good walk is a 'must' every day for both men and women. The fact that a woman is getting lots of exercise in the home does *not* compensate for an invigorating walk in the fresh air.

Some simple exercises for about ten minutes each day are very beneficial as they 'take out' some nervous tensions and strains and help to relax the sufferer.

Really hot baths should never be taken as they are very enervating. The water should be warm to tepid and afterwards the body should be rubbed briskly with a rough towel.

Rest plays a big part in the healing of jangled nerves. Getting to bed early and having a good night's sleep helps tremendously.

It is a very good thing to encourage people with nervous tension, etc., to take up an interesting hobby and to make social contacts; thinking of others does much to avoid introspection and depression and remember

'Laugh and the world laughs with you,
Weep and you weep alone'.

THERAPEUTIC INDEX

Chorea (St. Vitus's dance), Mistletoe.
Depression Avena sativa, Balm, Borage, Bugloss, Holy Thistle, Rosemary.
Grief, Borage, Sage.
Hysteria, Balm, Black Horehound, Catnep, Lady's Slipper, Lime Flowers, Mistletoe, Motherwort, Passion Flower, Rosemary, Scullcap.
Menopause, Motherwort, Passion Flower.
Neuralgia, Mistletoe, Passion Flower, Scullcap, Wood Betony.
Neuralgia of face, Hops
Nerve tonic, Avena Sativa, Avens, Hops, Lady's Slipper, Marjoram, Mistletoe, Valerian, Vervain, Wood Betony.
Nerves, relaxing, Balm.
Nerves, soothing, Balm, Black Cohosh, Catnep, Chamomile, Holy Thistle, Honey, Hops, Lime Flowers, Passion Flower, Scullcap, Valerian.
Nervousness, Catnep, Valerian, Vervain.
Nervous debility, Black Horehound, Catnep, Mistletoe, Valerian.
Nervous exhaustion, Avena Sativa, Honey, Sage, Vervain.
Nervous excitement, Black Cohosh.
Nervous headaches, Bugloss, Chamomile, Marjoram, Passion Flower, Rosemary, Scullcap, Valerian, Vervain, Wood Betony.
Nervous indigestion, Hops.
Nervous irritability, Lady's Slipper, Lime Flowers, Motherwort.
Nervous restlessness (during menopause), Passion Flower.
Nervous twitching, Scullcap.
Relaxing, Balm, Black Cohosh, Catnep, Lady's Slipper.
Restlessness, Lime Flowers, Scullcap.

Sleeplessness from jangled nerves, Balm, Black Cohosh, Honey, Lime Flowers, Passion Flower, Valerian.

Sleeplessness from nervous exhaustion, Avena Sativa, Scullcap, Vervain.

Soothing to the nerves, Balm, Black Cohosh, Catnep, Chamomile, Holy Thistle, Honey, Hops, Lime Flowers, Passion Flower, Scullcap, Valerian.

Soothing in nervous complaints of women, Chamomile, Motherwort.

Tension, Balm.